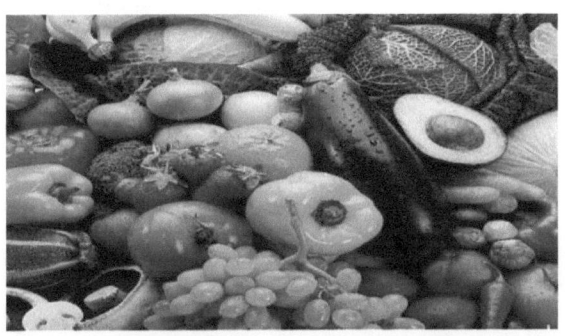

A GUIDE TO A HEALTHIER LIFESTYLE

Living Foods & Exotic Tastes

A GUIDE TO A HEALTHIER LIFESTYLE

Living Foods and Exotic Tastes

Published by Hunterschild Publishers 2013

ISBN: 978-1-30460-370-8

TABLE OF CONTENTS

Dedication

Acknowledgements

Disclaimer

Foreword

Introduction   11

Come With Me on a Walk through My Raw Food Journey   14

My Story – An Extract from My Journal 2009   16

My Lifestyle Change Launch Programme   19

The Starting Point   26

Some Juicy Tips   28

Exercise   30

An Example of My Dinner Plate   32

It's a Matter of Mind over Matter   34

My Raw Lifestyle   36

Transitioning to Raw Foods   38

Examples of Raw Foods   39

For my African Family   **43**

Vegetables and Their Health Benefits   **45**

Re-Emphasizing the Juicy Tips   **47**

Good to Know - Sleep   **50**

What I have learnt   **51**

Water   **52**

God gave me Children so I can send them on errands

    – A great Injustice   **57**

Shifting That Weight   **60**

My Why   **62**

Watch That Appetite – An Extract   **63**

Foods to Avoid   **65**

Body Odour   **66**

Some Natural Health Remedies   **67**

Is All You Eat Only Fruits and Vegetables   **69**

Recipes   **71**

Are You Still Eating Wheat? An Extract   **99**

Your Launch/Detox Programme   **104**

A Final Word   **106**

Next Steps   **108**

The Books that changed my way of thinking and helped me

on this journey   **109**

Short and Sharp Juicing Tips   **110**

Still not Sure?   **111**

Your notes   **112**

Dedication

This book is dedicated to my dear friend who became a sister OLUFUNKE KEHINDE MAKINDE-KAYOMA. ~ An Angel sent to me.

You were one of the reasons for this book.

I still clearly remember your voice saying "Sister Yetty, where is this your juicing book?"

You encouraged me on this healthy lifestyle journey, believed in me and tried out all my recipes.

You have gone to be with the Lord but you are constantly remembered.

Acknowledgements

This book has been in the oven for too long. It took spending five minutes with a new friend who asked me this question." Where's that book?" to reawaken my slumber.

My thanks go to my Father Almighty for sparing my life and allowing me to be a blessing to others through my own experience.

I would like to thank my Daddy, Revd. Canon Akande Odebiyi, and my wonderful step-mum, Mrs. Yemisi Odebiyi, for their prayers, support and also, for trusting me enough to try my juices and smoothies.

Thanks to my darling gifts from God, my best friends Omobosola, Moyosoluwa and Oluwatimilehin for allowing me those numerous "time outs" to do my thing including writing this book. I love you immensely.

To my mentor Nike Folarin, thank you for teaching me that I could eat and enjoy raw while incorporating Nigerian and African tastes.

To Temi, who held my hand and nudged me in the right direction, to **'wake up'** from my mini-slumber.

Thanks Chanda, my accountability partner, for those Tuesday afternoon accountability meetings.

Many thanks to Chief Mrs. Mosunmola Daramola for believing in me and always encouraging me to put all this into a book.

Olori Olufunke Lipede, my sister from another Father and Mother – thank you for your input during my research.

My mentor and online coach (now become sister), Elizabeth Horlemann. German - Kenyan, motivational speaker. For those words: "Yetty, if you do not publish that book, God will hold you accountable". Asante (Ki Swahili).

My proof readers, Tsola Abrahams, and my two daughters, thank you.

Pastor Yinka Dixon-Oludaiye, my cousin, sister and friend for that final push to get the book published, thank you.

I must not forget my big brother, Kunle Hamilton, President Shaddaiville Ministries, for teaching me to "release the Eagle in me", encouraging me to exchange mediocrity for excellence and also my Shaddaiville Leadership Academy Course mates UK 2009 set, who trusted me enough to try one of my smoothies after our final exams.

Finally, thanks to all my family (blood and not) and friends for their support and encouragement.

I love you all, thanks for being you and for being there.

Disclaimer

This book has been written based on my own personal experience.

I am not a medical person.

I am however learned, read a lot and ask lots of questions.

This book has been written in good faith and is been offered as an advice manual.

As a child I suffered from Asthma and Eczema. This conditions continued into my older years. I have however found that the lifestyle change embarked on after Cancer treatment helped alleviate some symptoms of these ailments.

The ideas and suggestions in the book in no way replace medical expertise.

Please do not stop taking your medication while using my suggestions without consulting your medical practitioner.

My Doctors were and are still aware of the progress I made while incorporating the lifestyle change. My medication has been adapted to suit my new lifestyle.

Also please note that some fruits and vegetables interfere with certain medications.

Please read the information slips on all your medications before embarking on Raw Juicing.

Having said this, bear in mind that the publishers of this book and I will take no responsibility for any loss or damages that might occur with respect to anyone who follows what I did and fails.

Foreword

I am most delighted and feel very honoured to write this
foreword to what is essentially a most useful and practical
health advice book of its kind.
The Author has poured herself out wholeheartedly,
truthfully, factually and with all sincerity and purpose, the
details of her personal experience through what I call 'a
journey of health'.

The advice from her rather 'rich' experience is aptly aided
with not just relevant books from various authors but also
from The Bible and its injunction (- not a surprise though
as she is a staunch practising Christian.)
The result is a special & robust health book which is
tailored to meet the needs of Africans but from which
people of other descents & races will benefit - leading to
life changes for the better.

I know for a fact that the Author is not medically trained
but I am amazed by her good grasp of the facts of
medicine & medical practice, with which she has
supported her arguments all through this book. Beyond
food, her advice regarding sleeping patterns, exercise,
water etc., are helpful, straight to the point and laid out in

simple understandable language - devoid of unnecessary medical jargon.

I personally know, for instance, some people (adults & kids) who do not drink water. They would do well to take a right cue from the advice in this book.

The depth and width of the content of the book encompass and adequately deal with such common problems e.g. being seen as 'anti-social' when out socialising; having snacks and the old time craving for 'swallow' or 'okele'.

The energy put in by the Author to write this book in order to share her personal health experience (confidentiality not spared) to enable help others possibly embark on the road to and enjoy a healthy lifestyle, is not just commendable but outright BRAVE.
I wholeheartedly recommend its reading to everyone out there who is conscious of the benefit of healthy living.

- Dr David 'Lai Soile.

Snr Partner, Gravesend Medical Practice

INTRODUCTION

It's easier to start this book giving a background story.

The background was that I was a normal working class wife and mother. Working, running my home and studying at the same time.

After abusing my body, it became run down and I was diagnosed with the C disease in 2005. By abusing my body I mean rushing around doing a lot of things – working, running my home, and standing at the kitchen worktop grabbing my meals on the rush and not really paying much attention to resting. So for a while my life stopped. My body no longer belonged to me. It belonged to the Cancer Specialists, the Oncologists, and finally the Plastic surgeons. While on this journey a darling Aunt suggested I tried the Hallelujah diet. We arranged a time when she would come to stay with me so we could start. That time however did not come.

After all the treatment, my body was tired and being unable to do a lot of things the weight piled on.

In January 2009, I attended an old girls meeting and six of my friends decided that we would look for ways to shift our "love handles". We set up a face book group and agreed to weigh in every Sunday morning.

A GUIDE TO A HEALTHIER LIFESTYLE

I decided to go all out and come up with ways to shift this fat. So, this is my story.

On the 11th of January 2009 I weighed in at 101kg and I was a size 20.

We weighed in a few times and then the novelty wore off. Life happened, other things got in the way. I however, decided to continue trying to find ways to lose the extra weight.

In the middle of January I came across a page on Facebook where the lady said she needed people to take a 28 day raw food challenge. Upon visiting the page, I found out it was being organised by a Nigerian. My first thought was "this lady would definitely understand the African taste". So I decided to try the raw food challenge. The first thing I had to do was to have juices and smoothies for my meals. The thought of this Raw Food business was a bit daunting but I decided to try it.

So on the 28th of January 2009, I added a couple of fruits and vegetables into my blender added water and voila...my first smoothie. It was a **scary looking green mix**. I was not sure if I could drink it. However, when I drank my first cup, I felt like oxygen had entered my body. I thought **"wow, this is the life".** I finished the full blender of smoothie in a couple of mouthfuls. My daughter looked at me in awesomeness not understanding that I could drink "that stuff".

A GUIDE TO A HEALTHIER LIFESTYLE

That was how my raw food experience was born.

I kept a record of what I ate and weighed myself every Sunday morning religiously.

By the time I attended Nike's "Reversing Diabetes in 30 days seminar" on the 28th of February I had lost 8 lbs. (3.63 kilograms) and was much fitter than I had in a long time. – That was only four weeks after I started incorporating raw foods into my diet.

From having a disabled badge and not being able to walk long distances, I was able to run up the stairs, go on long brisk walks without being out of breath; I thought I must be doing something right.

On the raw juice diet, I was losing 2lbs a week consistently. However what was most important for me was that I was not only getting my pre-cancer energy back, I even had more energy that I had ever had.

That is the reason for this book.

A GUIDE TO A HEALTHIER LIFESTYLE

COME WITH ME ON A WALK THROUGH MY RAW FOOD JOURNEY

It's easy for me to take you on my Raw Food journey from January 2009 to date as this is my true story. If you decide to try this challenge, I am confident you will benefit from it. I am not expecting you to become a 100% raw fooder, but you can at least aim for 75%. It is do-able.

Being the granddaughter of a hunter (Omo Odebiyi) and previously I could 'eat a whole cow', now I have limited my red beef intake to one small piece a week or none at all.

This book will be a recall of my journey on the Healthier lifestyle choice through Raw Foods whilst still enjoying my familiar traditional tastes. I will share extracts from my Journal which included whatever I ate.

You will also have recipes and ideas of meals, the health benefits of most fruits and vegetables. Tips to begin a healthy lifestyle change will also be included.

At this point I must say that if you are looking for a diet book, this is not a diet book but a book about a healthy lifestyle change. You'll understand more as your read.

So where do I start? The beginning I hear you say. The crux of the matter was that in the beginning I was overweight and was constantly tired. Within a few days of juicing, I was happier, lighter and my confidence increased.

I write from my experience. I am not a medical person but I read a lot, I am very inquisitive and love helping people and that is the "WHY" of this book.   I am also a firm believer of the saying "experience is the best teacher".

Jason Vale "the juice master" was one of my "mentors" on this journey. I am also aware that there are lots of books out there. Jason's book is my third bible following HALLELUJAH Diet by George Malkmus. The first and uttermost book - Bible, being the word of God.

Then God said "I give you every seed-bearing plant on the face of the whole earth and every tree that has fruit with seed in it. They shall be yours for food." Gen 1:29 (NIV).

This verse has been my inspiration. God's desire that we are allowed to eat the herbs and vegetables in the garden.....Eating foods in their natural state or at least in their "near natural, unadulterated state.

A GUIDE TO A HEALTHIER LIFESTYLE

MY STORY – An Extract from my Journal 2009

Following breast cancer treatment, I put on a lot of weight, going from a size 16 to size 22.

I decided in January 2009 together with a few friends to try and lose some weight and committed to weighing in every Sunday. We decided to help one another with any weight loss tips we found.

One of the tips included drinking two cups of water with fresh lemon first thing and also having breakfast and eating dinner as early as possible in the evening.

I lost a few pounds. However two weeks after I started watching what I was eating, I noticed that a friend on face book joined a group called "the raw food challenge". The challenge was to eliminate meats and most of our usual foods and go on a raw food diet eating fruits and vegetables and pulse and nuts.

My curiosity gave me the urge to try this and I stated raw juicing on the 28th of January, by the time I attended the seminar on the 28th of February, I had lost over 1 stone.

By having fruits and veg smoothies for breakfast and becoming 75% raw I was losing 2 lbs a week.

I was beginning to feel lighter and happier. My strength level increased. By the end of February I had gone from being always tired to having to check myself as my energy level increased.

The surprise for me was that in the first week of March I went upstairs and came back immediately. My daughter asked me what I had done. I said I went upstairs. She said "you RAN up the stairs 'mum' and ran back immediately". I had not been able to do this for years. I always have a rest when I get upstairs before considering coming down or usually ask one of the kids to run the errand for me.

On the raw foods, I am able to still enjoy my usual meals, including my "swallow". I enjoy Amala (Yam Flour) once a week with either raw Ewedu or raw Okro and a drop of stew. I have reduced my red meat intake to one small piece a week, if at all. I eat more fish, chicken.

I also noticed that my taste buds have changed. I enjoy lots of foods without salt. Mostly the seasoning I use is black pepper and some Knorr chicken or vegetable seasoning.

I could write a book, but on the raw foods life change I have lost over 10lbs and I am now able to get into size 16 clothes.

A GUIDE TO A HEALTHIER LIFESTYLE

I have gone from having a disabled badge as I was unable to walk long distances, to being able to take part in the Race 4 life. (An Annual 5 km charity walk to raise funds for Macmillan Cancer Care.) All thanks to moving onto raw foods. I don't see it as a diet, but see it as a lifestyle change.

It is all do-able, where there is a will, there is a way.

Benefits of raw juicing

1. Increased energy
2. Clearer skin
3. No headaches
4. No period pains
5. No constipation
6. More happiness as I am lighter
7. No hunger pangs.
8. I automatically sprint when walking and have to consciously slow myself down.
9. Improved sleep
10. No more puffy wrists and ankles.

Culled from my Journal March 2009

MY LIFESTYLE CHANGE PROGRAMME

It is likely that what worked for me might not work for you. However I want to implore you to at least have a go and be true to yourself. See if it works but you have to develop a "stick-to-it-ive-ness" attitude. No cheating.

For my launch Programme, I blended various fruits and vegetables together. My juicer, which had been bought about seven years previously, was tucked away in my under the stair cupboard. So many things prevented me access to the juicer, so I had to make do with my blender.

Before going on, I have to confess that I am not a fruit and veg person...yes, you read rightly. I am not the type of person who would sit down and eat any fruit or vegetable on a regular basis. I however found out that I was able to blend up to eleven or more fruits and vegetables and drink them as a refreshing smoothie. I hope that has not put you off.

This is a breakdown of my launch programme.

I will be taking you through a 6 month journey of my raw foods lifestyle. This is for you to get the picture of what worked for me. On the 11th of January 2009, I weighed in at **15 stones, 8lbs (101kg).** I believe that was my heaviest as at the previous Christmas, I could not eat much as I was very uncomfortable.

I started looking for ways to lose weight naturally, without using any diet pills or any of the tried and tested methods. On the 17th of January I came across Nike Coker's post on Facebook, asking for people to join her on a 28 day raw food challenge. She claimed she had gone from a size 20 to a size 14 and testified that this was due to juicing and eating raw. I became interested because she was African and I believed that she would understand my need better.

So I got ready and read a few examples of her smoothies online and decided to have a go. I had already started watching what I ate. I then decided to weigh myself first thing every Sunday morning. On the 25th of January I weighed in at **15st 8lbs (101 kg)**.

28th January 2009, I had my first smoothie.

1 x orange

1 x apple

1 x pear

A lot of raw spinach

A lot of kale.

A GUIDE TO A HEALTHIER LIFESTYLE

I chopped things up, added some water and put in my blender. (My 7 year old juicer was somewhere in the cupboard gathering dust). The blender was full, my daughter asked me if I was going to drink that green stuff and I said yes.

The first mouthful, I felt as if **oxygen** had been poured into my body…There was no going back.

So I began my raw foods lifestyle.

1st February, I weighed **15st 4lbs (97kg).** Something had to be working but it was early days yet.

8th February: **15st 2lbs (96kg)**. Okay, definitely something was working. I was so excited about my juicing; I was not keeping a record of my juices. However on the 10th of February, I started recording my juices on the calendar in my kitchen and also highlighted my favourites.

10th February, for breakfast, I had a juice made up of:

A handful of Spinach

A handful of Kale

Some green salad

1 x Banana

A GUIDE TO A HEALTHIER LIFESTYLE

1 x apple and green salad.

I did not record what I had for lunch or dinner.

11th February. For breakfast, my smoothie consisted of:

A handful of grapes

 2 broccoli florets

A handful of spinach

A handful of kale

Some green salad

1 x orange

½ apple

1 pear

½ banana.

I was so full; I skipped lunch and had a salad for dinner.

15th February I weighed **15st. (95kg).** I was so excited; I made a smoothie but did not record it.

16th February On waking, 2 large cups of warm water with fresh lemon. I read that lemon helps get rid of fat.

Breakfast:

A few pineapple chunks

A handful of spinach

A handful of kale

 1 orange

A kiwi fruit with some water.

Dinner: Sweet potato, salad and mackerel.

Tuesday 17th Breakfast:

Pineapple chunks

A handful of spinach

A handful of kale

1 x orange

1 x pear.

Dinner: Brown rice, raw spinach, and boiled chicken (without the skin).

Sunday 22nd February: **14st 9lbs (94kg).**

Saturday 28th February 2009. I attended the Raw Christian seminar hosted by Nike Coker. Today marked a turning

A GUIDE TO A HEALTHIER LIFESTYLE

point in my life. I walked for about 30 minutes without getting tired. I thought I must be doing something right. From having a disabled badge for not been able to walk far distances to this. I thought to myself "this is really working."

Sunday 1st March: **14st 8lbs (93kg).**

Sunday 8th March: **14st 6lbs (92kg).**

Sunday 15th March: **14st 5lbs (91kg).**

Sunday 22nd March: **14st 2lbs (90kg).**

Sunday 29th March: **14st (89kg).**

Sunday 5th & 12th April. I did not weigh in as I was in Nigeria and had no access to a scale. I was however juicing while I was in Lagos and watched what I ate.

Between January 2009 and December 2009, my weight loss was consistent as I continued on my healthy lifestyle choice options.

I have included the journey above in a diary form so you can see how do-able this lifestyle change is. Also to give you a truthful view of the starting point of my journey.

I continue to juice and adapt the way I cook my meals and also continued weighing myself every Sunday morning and in June I was at **80kg**.

A GUIDE TO A HEALTHIER LIFESTYLE

The chart below shows my weight loss from January 2009 to December 2009

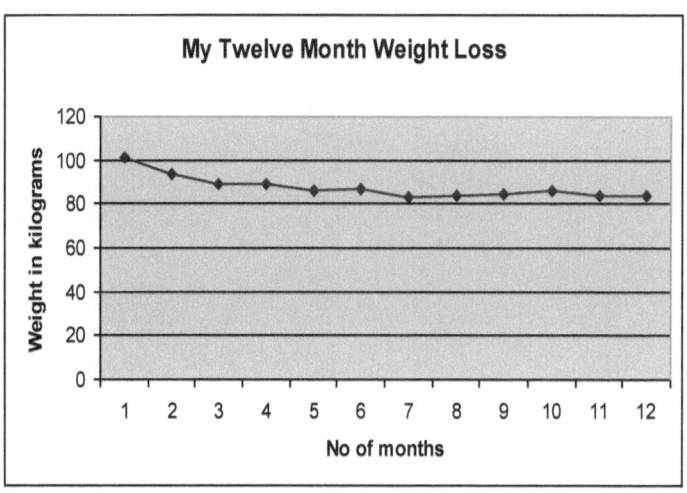

A GUIDE TO A HEALTHIER LIFESTYLE

THE STARTING POINT

Seeing you have read this far, I am going to assume that you are ready to make a lifestyle change. So here goes:

It is important that you educate your stomach that it does not rule your head. In fact, it is the other way round – **Your head should rule your stomach**. Every journey begins with the first step. Our first step is to think before you put anything in your mouth. Ask yourself these questions:

1. **What benefit will this food offer my body?**
2. **Am I hungry or am I thirsty?**

Weigh yourself. If you do not have a scale, go out and buy one or at least borrow one.

My starting point followed on from my conversation with my old school mates, we decided to lose some weight and tried to weigh in once a week. I doubt if any one followed through. However since January 2009, I weigh myself first thing on a Sunday morning. That way I know if there has been any weight loss or gain. I then plan my week based on my weight – whether I need to juice more to maintain my ideal weight or whether I need to lose some weight.

I have looked at the way we eat as Nigerians, Africans and I have come to the conclusion that most of what we eat is habit or tradition. If you disapprove, can you explain to me why anyone would want to put four or six pieces of assorted meats on their plate? Why would we eat our "swallows" so late in the night? Or why do we eat cow foot? What nutritional value is in cow foot?

Embarking on eating healthily is a life style change. You watch what you eat/ you think of what benefit will this food be to my body?

When the weight started dropping off me, effortlessly, I knew I was doing something right.

A GUIDE TO A HEALTHIER LIFESTYLE

SOME JUICY TIPS

Here are some juicy tips:

- Drink at least 8 glasses of water a day.
- Have 2 cups of water with fresh lemon/lime juice first thing in the morning.
- Fruit/vegetable smoothies

The best composition of your fresh fruits and vegetable smoothies or juicing really do matter.

My suggestion is 60% fruits and 40% vegetables. All fresh too.

The fruits help mask the taste of the vegetables. So I call the vegetables the medicine and the fruits the carrier.

- **Have your last meal by 6pm**. If later, have a very light meal Ogi (corn meal), Moin Moin (bean cakes) or just Efo riro (Spinach stew). (Eating late means your body works through the night to eliminate fats and if unable to do this, all is stored in the body).
- Eat lots of fruits in season
- Try to exercise for 1 hour 30 minutes a week. These can be spread throughout the week. Walks are good.

- Reduce food portions when you eat
- If you indulge and eat the 'bad' foods, start again the next day to eat healthy.
- Try to work on a seven day cycle, if you indulge in unhealthy foods during the week, try to detox and make up before the week is over – that way you won't scream when you next go on the scales.
- Drinking juicing/smoothies versus chewing – your body uses less energy to break down the juices/smoothies as opposed to chewed fruits/vegetables and this result in you being less tired. Your body immediately integrates the juices.

Tell your brain - "**I EAT TO LIVE, NOT LIVE TO EAT**".

If you can try a healthy lifestyle eating for 21 days, it will become a part of you. I have discovered that once the initial excess weight drops off within 5 to 6 months, you will stay the weight God wants you to be by just watching what you eat. It is doable.

EXERCISE

It would not be possible to write about a change in lifestyle choice without including exercising. It's part of the deal.

These tips worked for me. Also in January 2009, I was going to a "friendly" gym 3 or 4 times a week for a 25 minute session. I did not attend the normal gyms as I would have felt intimidated by those going to "pump iron". I also invested in a stepper which I used frequently at home.

Buying a mini-trampoline would be a very good investment. I could not imagine my 40 something year old self jumping on a trampoline. Once got one for my living room, I was hooked. I loved it. The mini-trampoline provides a "whole body" workout. It gets the heart pumping and you can exercise in the comfort of your home to music of your choice.

Whichever way you can, get at least 30 minutes of exercise each day. Walking, jogging, getting off the bus a couple of stops before your destination, parking your car a few yards away and walking the rest of the way are all forms of exercise.

I go for a walk with my accountability partner in the open air for 1 ½ to 2 hours each morning. It's a

A GUIDE TO A HEALTHIER LIFESTYLE

prayer/motivational walk. It's so nice to hear the birds in the wild around, breathing in fresh air before the cars come along to pollute the air.

It is likely that someone reading this book might not have access to a gym or there might be financial restrictions. You can still exercise in your own home. There are so many TV channels which include health programmes. You could buy a fitness video and watch and do this a couple of times a week.

You could go for walks, buy an exercise bicycle and use it for exercising NOT as a clothes hanger.

As I said before, you could even invest in a mini-trampoline. That ensures a full body workout.

Do something little. Start with the baby steps.

A GUIDE TO A HEALTHIER LIFESTYLE

AN EXAMPLE OF MY DINNER PLATE

This is an example of my dinner plate.

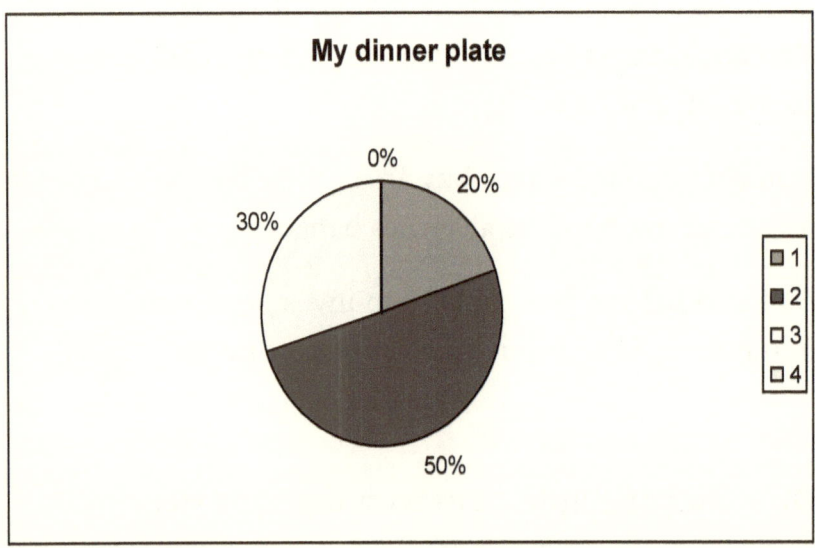

50% Raw vegetables (raw spinach or a salad)

30% Brown rice, Couscous or Bulgur wheat

20% Steamed Fish or boiled Chicken without the skin.

As I did not really like eating vegetables, I always ate my vegetables first and then the rice and chicken. That way I was almost full up with the raw vegetables.

An Example of one of my dinners:

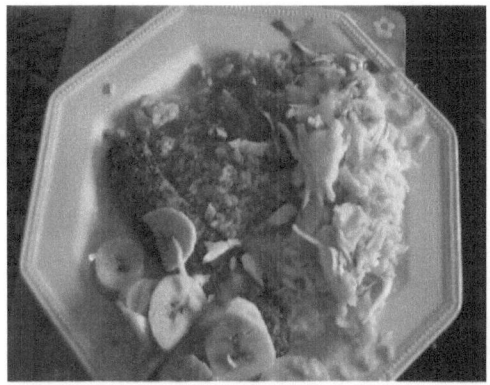

- Raw plantain

- One mackerel fillet

- Some brown rice

- Shredded cabbage

- A spoonful of stew

By the way I still cook "normal" foods for my family. The stew added to my plate above was the family stew and that consisted of:

Onions

Tomatoes

Red pepper

Sunflower oil

Seasonings

A GUIDE TO A HEALTHIER LIFESTYLE

IT'S A MATTER OF MIND OVER MATTER

I understand that starting on a healthy lifestyle option especially using the juicing and raw food method, could be a bit daunting but it is do-able. If you can stick at it, you'll see the results and become a happier and lighter person.

It gives me so much joy to do things myself instead of sending my children on errands. I am able to do more as I have more energy.

The Bible in Philippians 3:19 says "I can do all things through Christ who strengthens me" and that includes being in charge of your weight, your health etc.

Whatever you decide to do after reading this book, be it changing your eating habits, trying to lose some weight or just getting fitter, your heart has to be in it.

I have three young children in my household and that comes with its challenges. We always have what I call "a bad foods" including crisps, chocolates, ice-cream etc. around the house. I knew I had won the food battle when I was able to clear up their left-overs without any going in my mouth. I'm sure you can identify with that.

A GUIDE TO A HEALTHIER LIFESTYLE

I learnt that once you start on the raw food journey, your taste buds change and those sweet foods become TOO sweet for your palate.

Fruits and vegetables are expensive – a way round that is to grow your own. You don't even need a garden. You can grow in buckets.

A GUIDE TO A HEALTHIER LIFESTYLE

MY RAW LIFESTYLE

About Raw Foods

'Then God said, 'I give you every seed bearing plant on the face of the earth and every tree that has fruit with seed in it, they will be yours for food'. Genesis 1:29. **(NIV)**

It is about eating the following foods and basically not being cooked over 115°f - eating foods in their natural, unadulterated state.

Examples:

- Fresh fruits (organic, local, seasonal where possible)

- Fresh vegetables (organic, local, seasonal where possible)

- Nuts

- Seeds

- Super foods

- Sprouts, peas, beans and wholegrain

- Juices

- Smoothies

- Sea vegetables (Nori, Hyuki, Wakami)

Benefits of Raw Foods:

- You will have your natural, ideal body weight – without counting a single calorie!

- Great looking, shiny skin-glowing from the inside out.

- Pain-free period – menstruation can ago almost un-noticed

- You'll become more fertile (women only)

- Less illness

- More energy

- You'll start to reverse the signs of ageing

- You'll replace calorie counting with counting nutrients

- Any cellulite will start to fade or even totally disappear

- You'll nourish your body with food that is designed to be eaten.

- If you are currently sick, you will recover in faster time.

- Any disease within the body may start to repair

- You'll beat depression naturally

- You'll recover more quickly after exercise

- Your tummy will be flatter

- You'll live longer.

A GUIDE TO A HEALTHIER LIFESTYLE

TRANSITIONING TO RAW FOODS

◘ Take things slowly

◘ Cut down on your beverages (I went cold turkey and stopped drinking caffeine containing tea/coffee).

◘ Add juices/smoothies to your diet

◘ Add at least 2 raw ingredients to your cooked food. (e.g. Raw spinach or raw plantain)

◘ Start cutting down on red meat. (I have one piece of red meat a week or none at all).

◘ Have one raw meal day a week.

◘ Try a sample 100% raw challenge for a week. (There are lots of interesting recipes you can try).

◘ Keep a journal of your food. Yes – write down everything you eat. You will find some lovely recipes you'll want to repeat. (I write what I eat on the calendar in my kitchen.)

A GUIDE TO A HEALTHIER LIFESTYLE

EXAMPLES OF RAW FOODS

⊞ Juices

⊞ Smoothies

⊞ Salads (without the traditional dressings). I use homemade olive oil, balsamic vinegar and lemon dressing)

⊞ Raw veggie burger

⊞ Raw cookies

⊞ Milkshakes with almond milk

⊞ Raw chocolate

⊞ Raw ice cream

⊞ Raw spaghetti and spaghetti sauce

⊞ Fruit salad

⊞ Kuli Kuli (Nigerian delicacy made from Peanuts)

⊞ Soups

⊞ Milks

A GUIDE TO A HEALTHIER LIFESTYLE

- Foods not heated above 115°f (46°C) i.e. lesser cooking time)

(Recipes available on request)

- **DETOX**

- By juice fasting you cleanse and detoxify

- Day 2 and 3 are usually the most difficult as well as feeling hungry you may experience nausea or headaches. (I noticed this when I gave up on caffeine products especially tea).

EXAMPLES OF NIGERIAN RAW FOODS

- Raw Ewedu

- Raw Okro

- Raw Ugwu

- Sprouted beans

- All fruits/vegetables

To make the Raw Ewedu or Okro, wash them, cut them up and blend with boiling hot water. Your raw Ewedu or

Okro is ready. That's right! You do not cook it at all on the heat.

Examples of allowed meals on a raw diet:

Blended Quaker oats made as semolina/pounded yam

Smoothie of fruits with vegetables e.g. Spinach, Ugwu, Soko.

White meats e.g. chicken, fish.

EXAMPLE OF Raw diet Meals (including Nigerian style)

- ⌗ My healthy life e.g. 1 day.

- ⌗ On waking - 2 cups of warm water with few drops of fresh lemon or lime

- ⌗ Breakfast - fruit/vegetable smoothie

- ⌗ Lunch - salad with mackerel fillets or any fish

- ⌗ Dinner - spinach, rocket and watercress salad with avocado

- ⌗ Snacks - Almond, sultanas mixed seed including flax seed.

A GUIDE TO A HEALTHIER LIFESTYLE

◘ Once a week for lunch, I have Amala (yam or
plantain flour) or blended oats with Raw Okro –
Lady Fingers, (Abelmoschus Esculentus)or
Raw Ewedu (Corchorus Olitorius) or Molokhia
(Egyptian), a few spoonfuls of 'normal stew'
and a piece of chicken or fish).

A GUIDE TO A HEALTHIER LIFESTYLE

FOR MY AFRICAN FAMILY

Reduce your red meat intake with a view to cutting out completely. Instead eat more fish, chicken, turkey. COW foot (passionately called BOKOTO) is a no-no. No nutrients – just fat and eaten out of habit.

Moin-moin and boiled beans are very good foods that can aid the weight loss programme. However, enjoy your Ewa oloyin with no Palm oil. (Eat Ewa aganyin with very little or no sauce).

Raw Ewedu/ Okro. Wash very well with Milton, blend with boiling hot water. Serve.

If you cannot try this, only cook for 5 to 10 minutes.

If you are out, in order not to be antisocial, ask for Moin moin, chicken or fish and Efo riro. Yes, the Efo might have Palm oil in it, but if a small quantity is requested, there is no harm. Please note that chicken skin is very oily. Try to take the skin off.

SWALLOWS (Okele)

Amala and blended oats are the best. Other okeles can be taken but, in moderation. If you eat Pounded yam, it must definitely be before 6pm and preferably not more than once a week.

WATER is very important, drink water throughout the day. If you are in areas, where water cannot be trusted, carry your own bottled water around with you.

VEGETABLES AND THEIR HEALTH BENEFITS

As we age, it is important to know the benefits of the types of foods we put into our system. This will help us prevent disease and ailments.

So here are some health benefits of our fresh produce.

Beetroot – Beetroot is a good blood pressure buster. Drinking 500 ml of raw freshly made Beetroot juice can help lower blood pressure.

Broccoli – prevents high blood pressure; combats osteoporosis. Sulforaphane in broccoli helps to block cancer and is an anti-oxidant.

Carrots – carrot juice has anti-carcinogen properties. Thus helps prevent cancer and is believed to have cancer curing properties. Carrot juice has beta-carotene which is an antioxidant. It helps prevent cell degeneration and also slows down the ageing process. (By eating 1 carrot you only get 1% of the available beta-carotene, drinking a glass of freshly squeezed carrot juice; your system absorbs almost 100% beta-carotene.

Cauliflower – can prevent strokes and cancers.

Kale – prevents breast and ovarian cancer.

Okra/Okro – Soluble fibre helps to lower cholesterol, reducing risk of heart disease. Helps to keep the intestinal tract healthy, reducing the risk of some cancers, especially colon cancer. Okro helps prevent diabetes and constipation.

Spinach – helps stabilise blood sugars.

Swiss chard – one of the most powerful anti-cancer food

Ugwu – is a diuretic. Helps prevent high blood pressure and water retention.

RE–EMPHASIZING THE JUICY TIPS

Drink at least 8 glasses of water a day.

Have 2 cups of water with fresh lemon/lime juice first thing in the morning.

Drink fruit/vegetable smoothies.

Have your last meal by 6pm. If later, have a very light meal Ogi, Moin-moin or just Efo riro. (Eating late means your body works through the night to eliminate fats and if unable to do this, all is stored in the body).

Eat lots of fruits and vegetables in season.

Try to exercise for 1 hour 30 minutes a week. This time can be spread throughout the week. Walks are good.

If you indulge and eat the 'bad' foods, start again the next day to eat healthy.

Tell your brain "**I EAT TO LIVE, NOT LIVE TO EAT.**

If you can try a healthy lifestyle eating for 21 days, it will become a part of you. I have discovered that once the initial excess weight drops off within 5 to 6 months, you will stay the weight God wants you to be by just watching what you eat. It is doable.

A GUIDE TO A HEALTHIER LIFESTYLE

For those based in Africa, teach all those involved in food preparation in your home (including your children) to make a basic smoothie – pineapple chunks, orange, mango, Ugwu or Tete or any other green vegetable and 1 cup of water. So they can make it for you first thing in the morning.

These are just examples of the vegetables/fruit smoothies I have for breakfast or as my first meal (whenever that is), especially during times of fasting. You can adjust depending on your taste buds. Try and incorporate as many green leafy vegetables as you wish. (The greener the smoothie, the better).

I keep a diary of what I eat and here are some examples of my juices and smoothies.

- Carrots, kale, spinach, orange frozen berries and 1 or 2 cups of water.

- Spinach, kale, banana, apple, green salad, garlic, water.

- Grapes, broccoli, spinach, ginger, green salad, orange apple, pear banana.

- Pineapple, spinach, kale, orange, kiwi fruit.

- Carrots, broccoli, orange, pear, Italian salad, pineapple.

A GUIDE TO A HEALTHIER LIFESTYLE

- ½ pear, ½ orange, pineapple, spinach, kale, grapes ginger.

- Pineapple, mango, apple, Ugwu, spinach, kale.

- Mango, apple, spinach, ginger.

A GUIDE TO A HEALTHIER LIFESTYLE

GOOD TO KNOW

SLEEP

We cannot talk about healthy life options and losing weight using raw foods without talking about sleeping patterns.

Sleeping habits make a difference to our health and also weight loss.

From my own experience I know that those who sleep late have a tendency to wander into the kitchen for a late night snack and that snack could be anything. This then results in over eating as one would have had three meals that day and this could lead to the weight creeping up on one.

According to the National Health Service, "Good sleep is dream recipe to weight loss". Those who get around eight hours sleep a night and reduce their stress levels have doubled the chance of losing weight.

Those who have less than six hours sleep or more than eight hours per day are less likely to achieve weight loss than those who had between six and eight hours sleep. The results of the study also linked sleep patterns with obesity. However, this association does not mean that poor sleep causes obesity, or that healthy sleep patterns are a means of achieving weight loss. It is possible that underlying health problems are associated with poor sleep and obesity.

A GUIDE TO A HEALTHIER LIFESTYLE

WHAT I HAVE LEARNT

Flesh as Food

The diet appointed to man in the beginning did not include animal food. Not till after the flood, when every green thing on the earth had been destroyed, did man receive permission to eat flesh.   In choosing man's food in Eden, the Lord showed what the best diet was.   The best diet is one made up of raw foods, unprocessed foods and slightly cooked foods. For example, when we eat flesh i.e. red meats, we are receiving the vegetables second hand and also probably some of the diseases from these animals. Scientists have linked the consumption of red meats to many types of cancers.

For those who eat a lot of pork (pig), in any form, e.g. bacon, gammon, pork chops, spare ribs etc., it takes an average of **three months** for the deposits of these flesh to leave the body.

The non-elimination of these foods can result in headaches, other ailments and also fowl body odour.

If there is a family history of high cholesterol and high blood pressure, pork should be eliminated from the diet.

Also large quantities of red meat and processed foods should be avoided.

A GUIDE TO A HEALTHIER LIFESTYLE

WATER

Water is quite possibly the single most important thing in losing weight and keeping it off. Contrary to the belief of some, that water is fattening.

How 8 Glasses a Day Keeps Fat Away

(I was given this article at the Doctor prescribed gym I attended so many years ago. I don't even remember reading it neither did I start drinking 8 glasses of water a day until 2009.) It is good to share though)

HOW: it has been written that water, which most of us take for granted, may be one of the true permanent weight loss aids.

Water suppresses the appetite naturally and helps the body metabolise stored fat.

It has been found that a decrease in water intake will cause fat deposits to increase, while an increase in water intake can actually reduce fat deposits. This is because the kidneys cannot function properly without enough water. When the kidneys don't work to capacity, some of their load is dumped into the liver. One of the liver's primary functions is to metabolise stored fat into usable energy for the body. If however, the liver has to do some of the kidney's work; it can't operate at its full potential. As a result, it metabolises less fat and this fat remains stored in the body, and weight loss stops.

A GUIDE TO A HEALTHIER LIFESTYLE

Drinking enough water is the best treatment for fluid retention

When the body gets less water, it perceives this as a threat to survival and begins to hold on to every drop of water. Water is stored outside the cells and this shows up as swollen feet, legs and hands. Diuretics offer temporary solutions at best. They force out stored water along with some essential nutrients. The body perceives a threat and will replace the lost water at the first opportunity it gets, thereby allowing the condition to return quickly. The best way to overcome the problem with water retention is to give your body what it needs – plenty of water. Only then will water be released. If you have a constant problem with water retention, excess salt may be to blame. Your body will tolerate sodium only in a certain concentration. The more salt you eat, the more water your system retains to dilute it. Getting rid of unneeded salt is easy – **just drink more water**. As water is forced through the kidneys, it takes away excess sodium.

The overweight person needs more water than the thin one

Larger people have larger metabolic loads. Since we know that water is the key to fat metabolism, it follows that the overweight person needs more water.

(I remember my Dad telling my Step-Mum not to drink too much water as it was fattening. Now we know that it is the exact opposite).

Water helps to maintain proper muscle tone

This is done by giving muscles their natural ability to contract and by preventing dehydration. It also helps to prevent the sagging that usually follows weight loss- the shrinking cells are buoyed by water, which plumps the skin and leaves it clear, healthy and resilient.

Water helps rid the body of waste

During weight loss, the body has a lot more waste to get rid of, for example all that metabolised fat must be shed. Again, adequate water helps flush out the waste.

Water can help relieve constipation

When the body gets too little water, it siphons what is needed from internal sources and the colon is one primary source, resulting in constipation. However, when you drink enough water on a regular basis, the bowel function usually returns.

How much water is enough?

On average, a person should drink eight 8-ounce glasses every day. That's about 2 quarts (2.27 litres). However, the overweight person needs one additional glass for every 25 pounds of excess weight. The amount you drink should also increase if you exercise briskly or if the weather is hot and dry.

There is a school of thought that water should be preferably cold and that it is absorbed into the system more quickly than warm water. There is also a suggestion that drinking cold water can actually help burn calories. I drink either warm or cold water. (For those who say they don't like the taste of water, you can add a few drops of fresh lemon to your water or even fresh fruit slices and this will mask the "bland" taste). If you are an ulcer patient, please do not take fresh lemon or lime.

Results of Drinking water

When the body gets the water it needs to function optimally, its fluids are perfectly balanced. When this happens, you have reached the, breakthrough point". This means that the:

*Endocrine gland function improves

*Fluid retention is alleviated as stored water is lost

* Most fat is used as fuel because the liver is free to metabolise stored fat

* Natural thirst returns

* There is loss of hunger almost overnight

If you stop drinking enough water, your body fluids will be thrown out of balance again, and you may experience fluid retention, unexplained weight gain and loss of thirst. To remedy the situation you'll have to go back and force another, "breakthrough!"

GOD GAVE ME CHILDREN SO I CAN SEND THEM ON ERRANDS – A *Great Injustice.*

How many times have I heard my elders and my age mates make this statement? It's a great disservice to yourself. Get up and help yourself. Yes, God gave you children, but you have to move it.

The most important thing is that you get your body moving. Instead of calling the kids to get things for you, it is healthier to go up the stairs and get it yourself.

Be Active

It is never too late to get moving. Yes, I said to "get moving". No matter how old or young you are, you can benefit from physical activity. This could be so even if you have not been active for a long time. The journey of a thousand miles starts with the first step.

There are so many reasons for being active:

*Moving your body helps burn energy and also ensures that you keep a healthy weight

*Weight-bearing activities, such as walking, help strengthen the bones

*Regular physical activity helps keep your heart and lungs healthy

* Being active helps keep your blood pressure, blood cholesterol, and blood sugar normal

* For those who have trouble sleeping or loss of appetite, being active helps promote sleep and feelings of hunger.

Including physical activity in your daily routine can be both easy and enjoyable.

This might be a bit of a challenge to those of us, who feel that God gave us children to send them on errands. You are doing yourself a lot of injustice by sitting for so long on one spot and delegating duties.

It is important to aim for at least 30 minutes on most, if not all days. These activities can be split into three 10 minute spurts, or do it all at once.

Walking is one of the easiest and most convenient ways to be active. I go walking for at least 1 hour 5 days a week. First thing in the morning is very therapeutic and you get

A GUIDE TO A HEALTHIER LIFESTYLE

the fresh air. You have an added bonus if you live in the countryside – you tend to hear "the cock crow at dawn".

Other activities such as gardening, pushing the vacuum cleaner, using the stairs as opposed to the lift, carrying the shopping, walking instead of taking the car, would all count toward your daily activity.

It is important that you drink plain water when exercising, wear loose fitting clothes, and wear well-fitting sensible shoes when walking.

A GUIDE TO A HEALTHIER LIFESTYLE

SHIFTING THAT WEIGHT

If you think back to when you were younger, a lot of running around was done as children hardly sit still. The older we get, the lesser movements we make. The heavier we become, the lesser the movement we make. **Making a lifestyle change has to come from within.** Sometimes when people are given ideas on how to go about making a change, they reject it and this rejection could be due to various things including fear or pride.

You only have one life and the only person who can keep that life intact (apart from God) is yourself.

If you are overweight (and to 'thine own self' be true), this is the time to begin to take steps towards shedding that weight.

Being overweight can be likened to someone carrying a rucksack of books on one's back. Assume the rucksack has five books in it weighing 1 kilogram each. As you lose one book, the easier it becomes to carry the rucksack. Think of those books as your excess weight. As you consistently embark on a raw foods lifestyle change, your weight will drop down gradually. You will feel lighter and happier. Try it, if it doesn't work let me know.

A GUIDE TO A HEALTHIER LIFESTYLE

Did you know that one of the reasons why we do not notice that we have put on weight (except for the tight skirt or trousers), is because we live in our body, we see our body day in, day out.

One thing about the raw foods lifestyle is that when you start losing the weight, no part of your body will sag. This is because the raw (life) foods have the ability to repair the body as you consume them. Your cells regenerate and repair naturally. That is one of the advantages of a raw food choice as opposed to all other fad options out there.

The weight loss using the raw foods is a gradual but consistent loss. You can juice, eat healthy and lose any excess weight you want to shift.

MY WHY

All I have intended to achieve in putting this book together is to share my own weight loss experience. as well as sharing a healthier lifestyle option.

It would be nice to at least try to have a raw food day a week while on the transitional journey.

There are many books on the raw foods, but I have written this one especially for my African sisters and brothers.

Traditionally we eat out of habit and people are now suffering from health problems which end up being treated by the drugs which have so many side effects.

If we train ourselves to eat the things that are good for us, the body will repair itself, thereby preventing these illnesses.

Eating the right foods will also help in preventing most of these illnesses in the first instance.

A GUIDE TO A HEALTHIER LIFESTYLE

WATCH THAT APPETITE!

Culled from Open Heavens by **Pastor E.A. Adeboye** (General Overseer of the Redeemed Christian Church of God. A daily devotional 27th April 2011 (I couldn't help but share this)

"If you are a big eater, put a knife to your throat". (Prov. 23:2) NLT

Storing excess fat in the body leads to being overweight or obese, which in turn leads to high blood pressure, diabetes, stroke, sleep apnea, heart attack, heart failure, arteriosclerosis and other cardio-vascular diseases. **One major cause of obesity is over-eating or gluttony.** Food is good but excessive food is injurious to a good healthy life. Some people cannot stop their mouths whenever they see food. Even when their stomach is full, they continue to eat especially when "free food" is on offer. They are simply endangering their health! The bottom line is **moderation**. Proverbs 25:16 says, "Hast thou found honey? Eat as much as is sufficient for thee, lest thou be filled therewith and vomit it". We really need restraint when it comes to the quality and quantity of food we consume. Proverbs 24:13 confirms that honey is good

A GUIDE TO A HEALTHIER LIFESTYLE

for the body. It is a lot better than refined sugar if you are advanced in years. It is easier for your digestive system to break down the sugar in honey than that in refined sugar.

However, as good as honey is, it should be taken in moderation. Excess intake can lead to vomiting. This simply means that even when you are eating the right kind of healthy foods; it should be done in moderation. Gluttons are their own worst enemies. What they love the most ends up writing their obituaries! Is your excessive eating habit gradually sending you to an early grave? Stop it today! You have to be strict with yourself.

According to the above passage, if you love food too much, you must put a knife to your throat. In other words, exercise great restraint when you see food. Learn to say 'No' to offers of food. Learn to eat right. It is not only the quantity of food that matters but the quality also. Learn to fast. Sometimes, you can do a food fast that is not necessarily for spiritual blessings. Fasting is also good for the body's cleansing and metabolism. Remember that many are in the grave today, not because of any witch or wizard, but because of their appetite for food. Do not eat what will kill you, but would sustain your life.

A GUIDE TO A HEALTHIER LIFESTYLE

FOODS TO AVOID

There are so many types of food which would be good to avoid or at least eat in moderation. These include dairy products, wheat products and red meats.

Studies have shown that dairy products are not the solution to osteoporosis.

Try not to eat "like our great grandparents ate". They were more active than we are now. They did not have office jobs – they went to the farm and shifted any excess weight through manual labour.

After the age of thirty, it is advisable to change full fat milk for semi-skimmed milk. I do not take dairy products.

Also cut down or reduce your sugar and salt intake.

Try to avoid foods with a large quantity of fat. It is important to cut out Palm Oil completely or at least reduce the use in cooking.

Chicken skin has a large fat content. Remove the skin off your chicken – yes I know that is the part that has all the seasoning. It is healthier for you to take that skin off. Also avoid frying your chicken.

It is better to grill or bake your chicken and other foods instead of frying.

BODY ODOUR

You might not want to read this, but the more red meats, (flesh) we consume, the higher the tendency to have an offensive body odour. Why? You may ask me.

Look at this scenario: A person consumes a lot of carbohydrates and lots of red meats etc., with very little fresh vegetables or some 'over cooked' spinach/vegetable stews over a period of time. The foods are stored in the body and are not eliminated from the system. Due to the fact that the waste in the body is not completely eliminated, the body will start to produce bad body odour.

Literally speaking and please pardon me, **"The cow was already dead, we then cook it, fry it or roast it, further kill it by cooking it in stews and soups and then we consume it.....the odour emitted can be really offensive".**

To those who cannot do without eating meat, I would like to suggest that you begin reducing your intake of meats gradually and bulk up your intake of fresh or slightly cooked vegetables. Try it and see the result s you get. (No one even needs to know).

Please note: it is good to sweat, that is one of the reason why God put those pores on our bodies. It is the bad and **offensive odour** that is not allowed.

A GUIDE TO A HEALTHIER LIFESTYLE

NATURAL HEALTH REMEDIES

ARTHRITIS: Agbalumo - Chyrysophyllum Albidum (African Star Apple) can also be a good remedy for Arthritis. However a large amount of this would need to be consumed to obtain relief.

DIABETES: Bitter leaf helps reduce blood sugar. It also helps to repair the pancreas. Squeeze ten handfuls of fresh bitter leaf in 10 litres of water. Drink 2 glasses three times a day for one month. (Six glasses a day). Please note: Do not stop taking your regular medication.

DISEASED GUMS: Cucumber juice heals and refreshes diseased gums. Get a slice of cucumber and press it to the roof of your mouth with your tongue for a half minute, the phytochemicals will kill the bacteria in your mouth responsible for causing unpleasant breath.

GOUT & ARTHRITIS: As cucumber is an excellent source of silica it promotes joint health by strengthening the connective tissues. When mixed with carrot juice, cucumber can relieve gout and arthritis pain by lowering levels of the uric acid.

INSOMNIA: Banana can help eliminate depressive symptoms and also promote sleep. This is because banana contains Vitamin B6 and serotonin.

A GUIDE TO A HEALTHIER LIFESTYLE

MIGRAINE HEADACHES: On the onset of a migraine headache, wash red seedless grapes, put them in a blender and blend (adding no water). Drink the juice. This will alleviate the headache almost immediately.

PNEUMONIA: Squeeze the fresh bitter leaves (Vermonia Amygdalina) into water. Heat up the solution briefly so it is warm, not boiling. Drink one full glass three times a day. Continue for 4 weeks. A little honey can be added to preserve the solution.

SICKLE CELL ANAEMIA: Ugwu and other leafy greens like Spinach, Tete, Soko juiced together with apples can help to raise the haemoglobin levels and help prevent crises.

STOMACH ACHE: Chew tender bitter leaf like chewing gum, swallow the bitterness.

A GUIDE TO A HEALTHIER LIFESTYLE

IS ALL YOU EAT ONLY FRUITS AND VEGETABLES?

I have had so many people ask me if all I eat is fresh fruits and vegetables and the answer to that is NO!

The bulk of my foods consists of fresh raw fruits and vegetables but I still enjoy my familiar African traditional tastes. The difference is that I have adapted the way I prepare my meals.

I still eat my Okele e.g. Amala (yam Flour) and Oats (made like the swallow). I also eat Nigerian Beans, what I do is that I cook my beans and eat it bland, adding only onions when cooking. I remove my cooked beans before adding the oil and other ingredients to it for the family.

I also eat Moin Moin.

I have also substituted Olive Oil or Sunflower/corn oil for Palm Oil.

There are schools of thought that some of these oils are not healthy if they are heated and in order to reduce intake of such oils, I also cook with Coconut oil which is much healthier.

I swapped White rice for Brown Rice, Couscous and Bulgur Wheat. (Wheat kernel grain). Bulgur has fewer calories, less fat and more than twice the fibre than in Brown rice

I eat white meats like Fish, Chicken, Turkey without the skin.

If I am unable to eat a raw food, I ensure I have a portion of a raw food on my plate e.g. raw plantain, when I fry Dodo (Fried Plantain) for my family, or a fresh salad. I also sometimes just grate a couple of carrots and add to my plate or it could even be fresh washed uncooked Spinach.

I have a sweet tooth and eat the raw snacks sometimes.

After the detox programme and after I came to my ideal weight, I sometimes indulge in what I call "bad foods" but I have been able to watch my weight by juicing and eating the right foods within my week.

In order for the healthy eating to work, please do not deny yourself of things you like to eat – the idea is to eat things in moderation and think before you eat.

A GUIDE TO A HEALTHIER LIFESTYLE

RECIPES

In this section, I will include some of the recipes that worked for me and that I really enjoyed.

GREEN SMOOTHIES

A green smoothie means that the smoothie has leafy greens in it. For example, a basic green smoothie would comprise of mango, apple, and a handful of Spinach. The mango and the apple mask the taste of the Spinach and make it more palatable. After a while, your taste buds get used to it. I remember the first time I added Ugwu as my leafy green. It was a very harsh taste, but my taste buds are now used to it. The greens have high levels of many nutrients and are low in calories. When you mix the leafy green with the fruit the mixture reduces the amount of calories in the smoothie.

A GUIDE TO A HEALTHIER LIFESTYLE

SMOOTHIES AND JUICES

A Basic Smoothie (just to get you into the groove of juicing)

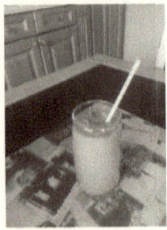

1 apple

1 mango

A handful of spinach or Ugwu or any leafy green

Optional a little cut of fresh ginger.

Put all ingredients in a blender, add 2 cups of water, blend and enjoy!

JUICES

PINEAPPLE & BEETROOT MEDLEY

This is one of my favourites.

1 beetroot

1 apple

6 pineapple chunks

½ celery

Handful of spinach

3 carrots

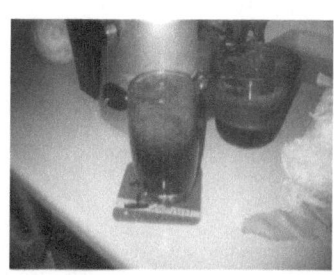

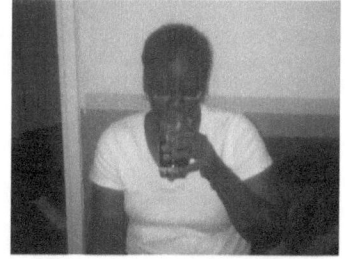

Wash all these fresh fruits/vegetables, cut and place into your juicer and add ice cubes (if you wish) and drink. This is so refreshing it got an A* on my calendar.

Health benefits:

Beetroot can help detox the liver, assist in eliminating toxins and also avoiding a build-up of fatty deposits. Beetroot can help prevent strokes and heart attacks. Researchers at Bart's Hospital (London) and the London School of Medicine found that **drinking 500ml of**

A GUIDE TO A HEALTHIER LIFESTYLE

beetroot juice a day can significantly reduce high blood pressure over 24 hours after drinking.

(Whatever you do, if you are on medication, please do not stop taking your medication while juicing. If you doctor asks you what you are doing that has aided a decrease in the high BP, please let him know. You will find that your doctor will encourage you to continue doing whatever you are doing that is making a POSITIVE difference to your health).

Beetroot is also packed with both Vitamin C and iron, which are wonderful for your body. Vitamin C also helps increase the absorption of iron. Since Vitamin C is water soluble, which means you lose a lot of this from cooking, the easiest way to benefit from this is to eat or juice raw beetroot.

The roots are also a good source of other vitamins and minerals which include folic acid, phosphorous, magnesium and B6.

Beetroot is also an immune booster. It helps to regenerate your blood cells.

Apples have many benefits. These include the prevention of many cancers, Alzheimer's disease. The pectin in apples supplies galacuturonic acid to the body which lowers the body's need for insulin and may help in the management of diabetes. Apples can also help to assist weight loss.

A GUIDE TO A HEALTHIER LIFESTYLE

Pineapple has too many health benefits which include helping with inflammations; it can be used to manage pain associated with arthritis. Pineapple helps to relieve heartburn, indigestion, treats nausea. It helps to reduce sinus inflammations, bronchitis and helps reduce cough and mucus. The Bromelain in pineapple may help increase the body's ability to naturally kill tumours.

Celery leaves are high in Vitamins A. The stems are full of Vitamins B1, B2, B6 and C. these supply potassium, folic acid, calcium, magnesium, iron and sodium. Celery helps lower blood pressure, prevents cancer, and is a good diuretic. Helps in weight loss and can also assist in the breakdown of urinary and gall bladder stones.

Spinach is rich in vitamins A & C. helps to lower blood pressure, helps control cancer. Protects against heart disease and prevents cataracts.

Carrots are also high in vitamins. Help to control blood sugars, reduce the blood pressure. This is a good treatment for strokes; an energy booster.

A GUIDE TO A HEALTHIER LIFESTYLE

SPINACH GUINNESS

This juice looks like stout, Guinness…

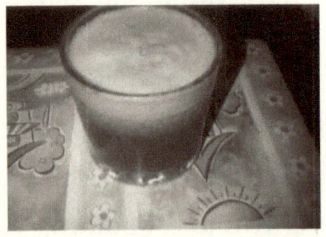

2 handfuls of baby spinach

¼ pineapple

¼ cucumber

1 medium carrot

1/3 lemon, peeled

Ice

Juice the spinach, pineapple, cucumber, carrot and lemon. Then add ice cubes.

Health Benefits: This juice is known to be rich in iron and will benefit you more than 10 pints of Guinness.

AVOCADO 'n' PINEAPPLE PICK ME UP

This is another favourite of mine. It's the first juice my daughter agreed to have more after she tasted some. It's usually requested and a taste will be the judge of that. I now have to hide my smoothie once it's made.

½ a medium pineapple

½ ripe avocado (organic is best).

1 peeled lime

Ice cubes.

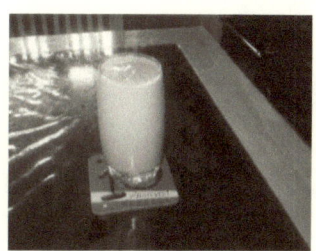

Put the avocado flesh and ice cubes in a blender.

Juice the pineapple and lime.

Add the juice into the blender and blend until smooth.

If you do not have a juicer, place all the produce in a blender and blend until smooth.

Some people believe that pineapples and avocados are fattening but this is incorrect. From my own experience if this were true, my weight loss would not have happened as I use pineapples as a base for my juices/smoothies also every day since March 2009. Also, according to the Guinness book of records, Avocadoes are the world's most nutritious fruits.

Health benefits: Pineapple is anti-inflammatory and its enzymes aid digestion of protein. Good for arthritis. Also helps break down mucus, so good for asthma sufferers.

CARROT REVITALIZER

3 carrots

2 apples

1 orange

Scrub and trim the carrots and quarter the apples. Peel the orange (leaving some of the pitch on) and cut into rough segments.

Juice the carrots and the fruit, pour into a glass and serve immediately.

This powerful drink nourishes and stimulates the system. It is a lively health-giving drink.

CITRUS SPARKLE

1 pink grapefruit

1 orange

30ml/2 tsps. freshly squeezed lemon juice

Cut the pink grapefruit and orange in half and squeeze out the juice in a juicer or using a citrus fruit squeezer.

Pour the juice into a glass, stir in 75ml lemon juice and serve immediately.

Health benefits:

Studies show that grapefruit can aid in weight loss. It is low in sodium but high in fat burning enzymes. It is a powerful antioxidant. Grapefruit contains vitamins C, A and lycopene. These antioxidants help to rid the body of free radicals and excessive oxidisation that can cause cancers. Lycopene which is a carotenoid found in the red/pink hues help prevent occurrence of tumours and cancers.

Grapefruits can also help to prevent or lessen the symptoms of arthritis. It can also help to reduce cholesterol.

However if you are on medication, please inform your health practitioner before embarking on consuming, lots of grapefruit juice as these could interfere with some medication. Extra care should be taken especially when on high blood pressure medications and Statins.

A GUIDE TO A HEALTHIER LIFESTYLE

HONEY AND WATERMELON TONIC

1 watermelon

1 litre/1 ¾ pints /4 cups chilled still mineral water

2 limes

Clear honey, to taste (optional)

Cut the watermelon flesh into chunks, remove the skin and discard the seeds. Place in a large bowl, pour the chilled water over wand leave to stand for 10 minutes.

Pour the mixture into a large sieve placed over a bowl. Using a wooden spoon, press gently on the fruit to extract all the liquid.

Stir in the lime juice and sweeten to taste with honey, if you like. Pour into glasses and serve.

Health benefits:

Watermelons are a great source of Vitamins A, C & B6. Vitamin A helps maintain eye health and is an antioxidant. Vitamin C helps heal wounds, prevents cell damage, strengthens immunity, while Vitamin B6 helps convert protein to energy. Watermelon has a large concentration of lycopene - an antioxidant, which helps in fighting heart disease and several types of cancers especially prostate cancer.

A GUIDE TO A HEALTHIER LIFESTYLE

CARROT & PINEAPPLE TWIST

1 apple

2 carrots

¼ pineapple

¼ lemon with skin on

Handful spinach

Ice

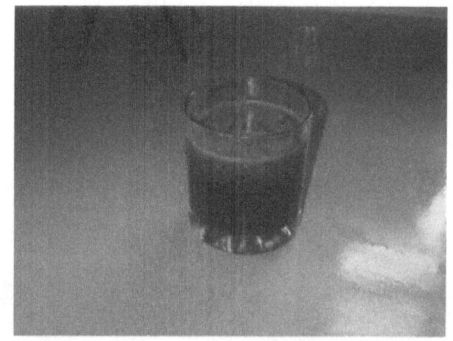

Place all the produce into a juicer or a blender. Juice and pour over the ice.

FRUITY KALE

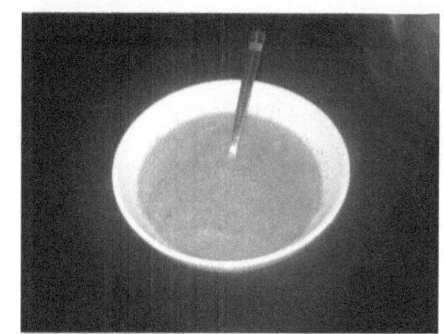

1 apple

I banana

1 pear

2 handfuls of Kale

1 rib celery

1 cup of water

A GUIDE TO A HEALTHIER LIFESTYLE

Cut all the produce into small sizes, put inside the blender with the water. Blend until very smooth. Pour into a cereal bowl and drink with a spoon. You could also pour it into a glass and enjoy. (I prefer eating it as a cereal. I get a more satisfying feeling).

SOUPS/STEWS

I love making these soups because they are ready in no time.

SWEET POTATO, COCONUT & CHILLI SOUP (An African Twist)

2 medium sweet potatoes

1 small red chilli, seeds removed if you want

1 small red onion

1 tablespoon of olive oil

1 can of half-fat coconut milk

A GUIDE TO A HEALTHIER LIFESTYLE

Method:

Peel the sweet potatoes and chop into small chunks.

Chop the chilli and spring onions or onions into small slices.

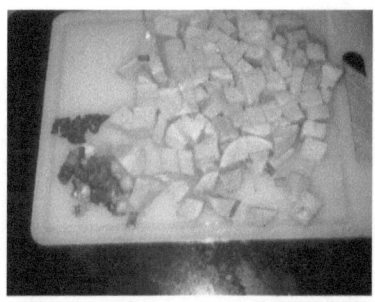

Heat the oil in a large saucepan and add the sweet potatoes, chilli and onion.

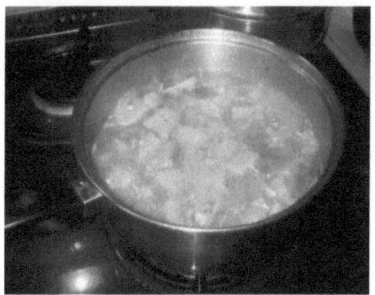

Gently sweat the vegetables over a medium heat for 15 minutes then add the coconut milk and simmer for 10 minutes.

A GUIDE TO A HEALTHIER LIFESTYLE

Remove from the heat and using a blender blend the soup until smooth.

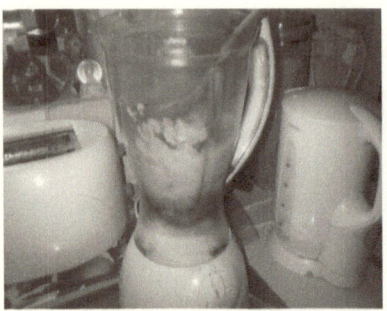

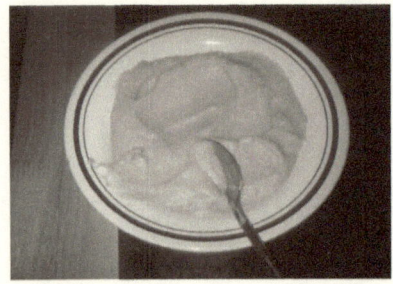

Pour into a bowl and enjoy.

Health benefits: The sweet potatoes and onions together help to stabilise blood sugar levels. The onions can help lower chances of colon cancer and are beneficial to bone health. They are also anti-inflammatory and help lower high blood pressure and cholesterol. The sweet potatoes are a good source of beta-carotene and Vitamin C. Together these antioxidants work in the body to eliminate free radicals and therefore help prevent disease.

A GUIDE TO A HEALTHIER LIFESTYLE

CARROT and BUTTERNUT SQUASH SOUP (one of my favourites)

3 medium carrots

½ Butternut Squash

1 small red onion

1 stock cube (Knorr)

1 tbsp. Olive oil

Black pepper

METHOD

Remove the skin of the butternut squash, carrots and red onion. Chop the vegetables into small chunks.

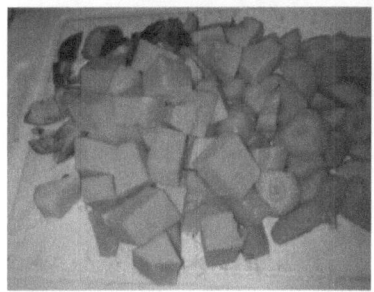

Dissolve the Knorr cube in 1 pint (570ml) of boiling water.

Heat the oil in a large saucepan, add all the vegetables and season with the black pepper.

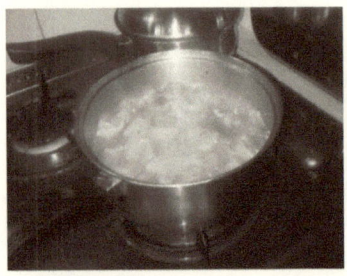 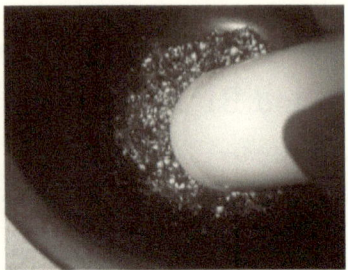

Cover the saucepan and sweat gently over a medium heat for 15 minutes, stirring occasionally.

Add the Knorr stock and boil for 10 minutes.

Remove from the heat and pour into a blender. Blend until smooth.

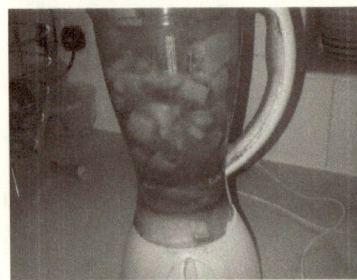 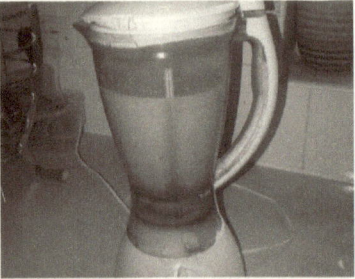

If you prefer to have chunks in your soup, do not blend too fine.

Your soup is ready to eat. Pour into a bowl and dinner is served.

A GUIDE TO A HEALTHIER LIFESTYLE

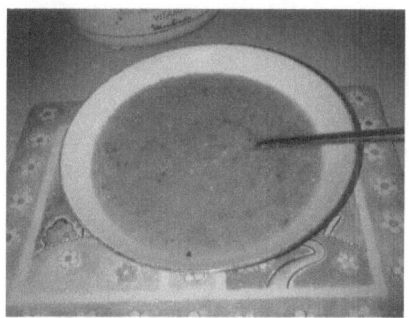

Health benefits:

Both the carrots and the butternut Squash have beta-carotene which are powerful antioxidant and anti-inflammatory properties.

These protect against cardiovascular disease and strokes. Also help protect against cancer.

A GUIDE TO A HEALTHIER LIFESTYLE

EFO RIRO (Vegetable Stew)

Ingredients

2kg/4lbs fresh spinach/soko/Tete/ Ugwu

250g dry fish/stock fish

250g smoked turkey

225g/8oz ground crayfish

225g/8oz fresh pepper or 2 Rodo (depending on how hot you like your stew)

500g/1lb fresh tomatoes/ 2 tins chopped tomatoes

2 medium onions

190 ml/6 fl oz. Olive oil/ corn oil/sunflower oil

1 teaspoon Iru (locust bean/carob bean) chopped or blended

1 pint stock or water

2 Maggi Keri or Knorr cubes

A tiny pinch of salt (optional)

PREPARATION

Chop the dry fish, stock fish and smoked turkey into small pieces.

Wash the Spinach, Tete, Soko or Ugwu thoroughly a couple of times in water. Cut into medium pieces.

METHOD

Heat the oil in large saucepan. Add the blended vegetables to the oil and season with the Maggi Kerri or Knorr cubes. Boil for 10 minutes. Add the Iru (locust bean), dry fish, stock fish and smoked turkey pieces. Simmer for another 5 minutes, and then add the choice of your vegetables or mixture to the pot. Simmer for 10 minutes, check your seasoning and serve, Yes, I said 5 minutes and your Efo riro (healthy style) is ready.

PLEASE NOTE: I do not blanch the vegetables prior in hot water as these removes all the nutrients. I only cook my healthy Efo riro for a maximum of 20 minutes start to finish. This ensures that all the nutrients are locked in. Your vegetables are still green looking and taste fresh.

Efo riro – It is good to substitute Palm oil for vegetable of sunflower/corn oil. You do not need the extra cholesterol in the Palm oil.

Also try not to overcook your vegetables. My Efo riro is cooked in less than 20 minutes – yes 20 minutes from start to finish. Reduce your chilli pepper intake. Once the Pepper, tomatoes and onions are blended and cooked, season with dry fish, Cray fish etc. and add the washed green vegetables direct to the tomatoes. Do not braise the vegetables in hot water first as we do. By doing that most of the nutrients in the Efo are lost.

A GUIDE TO A HEALTHIER LIFESTYLE

This now brings me to the issue of swallow (Okeles). I know most Africans, especially Nigerians love their Okele. When embarking on a healthy lifestyle option, it is advisable to eliminate, if not reduce the amount of heavy swallow foods we eat. Things like Iyan (pounded yam) or Eba (cassava) are no go areas. If however, you decide to continue eating such foods, they must be eaten in moderation. The reason is these foods take a long time to leave our system and thereby slow down the metabolism. "I have been eating these foods forever" (I hear you say). Yes you have, but what are the long term consequences of eating these foods without eliminating them from the system. Those familiar diseases we end up with in our older ages – high blood pressure, diabetes, heart attacks, cancer etc.

I also hear you say, "Our fore fathers ate these meals, prepared the traditional way and they lived to ripe old ages". Again, yes I agree, but our forefathers would eat Eba or Pounded yam and walk so many miles to the farm to do hard labour farming in the hot sun. We now drive our cars to work, sit at computers all day, come home, sit in front of the television or computer, eat the heavy foods and go to bed. That is if we do not fall asleep in front of the televisions. The only form of exercise some people do is the walk from the front door to the car and from the car to their office desk.

A GUIDE TO A HEALTHIER LIFESTYLE

My suggestions for Okeles (swallow) are only two types are allowed and also in moderation. These are Amala (Yam Flour) and Quaker oats. Yes, you read right, Quaker oats. I recommend Amala because it is light and digests easily and quicker than others. Quaker oats is good because of the nutritional value in oats and also due to the fact that it digests easily. Oats are also very good for the heart.

QUAKER OATS (swallow)

1 cup of Quaker Oats

1 cup of cold water.

METHOD

Pour the Quaker Oats into a blender, add the water.

Blend until smooth.

Pour the blender contents into a saucepan with a handle.

Bring to the boil, stirring with a wooden spoon.

Continue to turn until firm.

Turn onto a plate add Efo riro or another stew and enjoy.

Health benefits: Oats lower risk of developing heart disease; promotes feeling of fullness thereby helping in weight management. Helps promote a regular and healthy digestive system. Reduces the risk of cancer and promotes healthy blood pressure.

OATS/OATMEAL PANCAKES

Here's the recipe:

8 spoons Quaker oats, (Or other brand)

1 egg

Some sweetener (I use Agave nectar)

1 small cup of water, milk, or Soya milk or Rice milk

1 spoon Flaxseed (optional but very healthy) olive oil.

Put all ingredients except the olive oil in your blender. Blend to a paste. If too watery add some more oats. You get the pancake consistency.

Fry as you would pancakes.

Optional add cinnamon, or vanilla essence.

CAULIFLOWER RICE

1 head cauliflower (or however much you want)

To make this dish the most easily and to have it come out the best, three pieces of equipment are very helpful:

A food processor

A microwave

A covered (or fairly tightly coverable) microwave-safe dish

A GUIDE TO A HEALTHIER LIFESTYLE

METHOD

Process fresh cauliflower until it is the size of rice, either using the plain steel blade or the shredder blade. Alternatively, you can shred it with a hand-held grater, or even use a knife, if you have the dexterity to chop it up VERY finely.

Microwave it in a covered dish. DO NOT ADD WATER. Cauliflower absorbs water like crazy and the granules will become gummy. To keep it fluffy, just let the moisture in the cauliflower do its work.

Serve with stew of your choice.

Health Benefits: Another excellent source of vitamin C and manganese. Great antioxidant, helps in cancer prevention; Good detoxifier and reduces inflammation.

I understand that I have not covered all the recipes we have in the African diet. That would mean writing another book. **The purpose of this book is to give a background so that we can start thinking about adapting the traditional cooking methods to a healthier choice.**

I would like you to start thinking of eliminating or at least reducing the ingredients that are of no benefit to our health. Examples are: substituting corn or sunflower oil for Palm Oil or using Olive oil instead of sunflower oil, removing peanut butter from our cooking.

SNACKS

You will find here a few snacks which are allowed on the raw foods journey. While out and about, I have cut up pieces of carrots and a couple of fruits with me. These would keep the hunger prangs at bay and also prevent you from reaching for that chocolate bar.

For those with sweet tooth, a mixture of almonds, currants and mixed seeds are also good to have handy. The almonds are the carbohydrate, the seeds – the protein and the currants serve as the sugar.

I will also include some sweet snacks for those who cannot do without the sugar rush.

CHOCOLATE ICE-CREAM

1 ¾ cups cashews or pieces

1 ¾ cups water (preferably filtered)

1 cup Maple syrup

2 tbsp. vanilla flavour

¼ tsp. almond flavour

½ cup unsweetened cocoa or cacao powder.

METHOD

Combine all ingredients in a blender, pour into a container and freeze.

RAW ICE-CREAM

2 Vanilla beans

2 cups cashews or pieces

2 cups filtered water

1 cup maple syrup

METHOD

Grind the vanilla beans in a blender, add other ingredients into blender.

Pour into ice-cream tubs and freeze.

CRUMBLY NUT SQUARES

Tools: Food processor, greaseproof paper, baking tray.

65g Almonds

65g Brazil nuts

65g Raisins

65g Dates

¼ tsp. of Cinnamon

Pinch of Coriander

A GUIDE TO A HEALTHIER LIFESTYLE

METHOD

Blend all ingredients in a food processor. Press out on to a baking tray lined with greaseproof paper.

Chill until the mixture has formed a little. Then cut into squares and enjoy.

Please note: I did not forget…none of these go into the oven. They are raw sweets.

CHOCOLATE SWEETIES (recipe makes 8 sweets)

Tools: Food processor, biscuits cutter, rolling pin.

125g Cashew nuts

65g dates

65g Raisins

1 tbsp. cacao powder

1 tbsp. carob powder

METHOD

Blend all ingredients in the food processor until dough is formed. Roll on flat surface and cut out rounds using the cutter.

Ready to eat – Enjoy.

GOJI BISCUITS

Makes 10 biscuits

Tools: Food processor, rolling pin, biscuits cutter

100g Almonds

75g Cashews

65g dried Dates

65g Raisins

65g Goji berries

40g Lucuma (available from Health Food shops)

Put all the ingredients in the food processor and blend until makes dough.

Roll out dough on a flat surface and cut out little round shapes using the biscuit cutter.

ENJOY.

RAW CHOCOLATE BOMBS (My favourite)

125g Almonds

125g dates

125g Raisins

80g raw Cacao powder

Put all the ingredients into a food processor, blend until a dough forms.

Take little spoonfuls and using your hands, roll into little chocolate balls.

Store them in a container and enjoy.

I hope you enjoy these recipes as you begin the healthy raw lifestyle change.

Your feedback is always welcome.

A GUIDE TO A HEALTHIER LIFESTYLE

ARE YOU STILL EATING WHEAT?

Another Extract – Author unknown

My people, are you still eating wheat? Please think again. READ this:

I saw this online, and I decided to share it.

Wheat is now the preferred swallow meal for many Nigerian families particularly in the urban centres. Sadly too, some rural dwellers have hooked to the fad that wheat is a "healthy" food. Early this year, a middle-aged man from Ekiti State (Nigeria) came to my office for solution to his health challenges – diabetes and high blood pressure. Upon enquiry on his diet, he said wheat was his major meal daily. According to him, virtually all the civil servants working at the state and local governments in Ekiti State also eat wheat as their regular meal. In fact, he said those that are not eating wheat particularly in the state capital could not afford it, but not due to knowledge of its harm to health. What an irony? Otherwise, how do we explain the preference of wheat to pounded yam, which the Ekiti people have been eating for good health and vitality centuries back?

The prevalent consumption of wheat across the country has clearly shown that in the absence of knowledge, people can accept poison as therapy. After all, wheat is the first choice food for diabetics on the strength of doctors' advice. Nationwide, wheat has overshadowed yam flour and other starchy foods that are peculiar to our culinary culture in Nigeria. Unfortunately, this is one dietary change that may prove suicidal for many people given the inseparable linkage of diet to health or ill health. Though wheat, like other grains, is rich in fibre and some other nutrients, it is one food anybody that desires wellness and long life should be kept at arm's length. Why? There are three inherent dangers in the chemistry of wheat that make it a classic destroyer of health. I call them the downsides of wheat.

Wheat contains gluten – a protein that causes inflammation, a systemic process that has harmful effects across all the organ systems in the body including the brain, heart, joints, eyes and digestive tract. As a matter of fact, inflammation does not only precede all degenerative diseases like diabetes, cancer, stroke, glaucoma, arthritis and Parkinson's disease, but also fuels their insidious progression. A review paper in the New England Journal of Medicine listed 55 diseases that can be caused by eating gluten-containing foods. The diseases include osteoporosis, anemia, cancer, canker sores, fatigue, rheumatoid arthritis and multiple sclerosis. The paper also linked gluten to many psychiatric and neurological diseases including depression, schizophrenia, dementia, nerve damage, epilepsy and autism. The paper concluded that there are 120 or more diseases associated with eating foods that contain gluten. Dr. Joseph A. Murray, MD states that he is surprised how often gluten affects the

A GUIDE TO A HEALTHIER LIFESTYLE

brain. Another study by Dr. J. Robert Cade, MD of the University of Florida showed that people with autism and schizophrenia have high level of peptides in their urine. These peptides, according to Dr. Cade, come from casein (protein in milk and other dairy products) and gliadin and gluten in wheat, barley, oats and rye.

Another study of 30,000 patients analyzed from 1969 - 2008 reported in the journal of the American Medical Association found that people diagnosed with gluten-sensitivity had a higher risk of death from cancer and heart disease than the normal population.

Worse still, the bulk of wheat being consumed in the country is the American hybrid strain, which has much higher gluten content than the European wheat.

The second inherent danger in the chemistry of wheat is its high Glycemic Index GI. Glycemic Index is a scale that ranks carbohydrate rich foods by how much they raise blood sugar level compared to low glycemic foods. Wheat has GI of 71 compared to yam and sweet potato with GI of 49 and 54 respectively. Invariably, eating food with high GI like wheat regularly promotes weight gain and makes diabetes intractable. **According to Dr. Mark Hyman, MD "wheat is a major contributor to obesity, diabetes, cancer, dementia, depression and many modern ills." If one may ask, what is the**

A GUIDE TO A HEALTHIER LIFESTYLE

science behind the recommendation of wheat as a meal to fight high blood sugar?

Also, many people do not know that wheat, which is being promoted as a "healthy" food, is one of the most acid-forming foods. What are the health implications of eating acid forming foods? Wheat and other acid-forming foods lower the body pH and deplete oxygen level in the cells and tissues, which is the primary cause of all diseases. In other words, if wheat causes low pH that triggers diseases, eating wheat and its products is akin to adding fuel to fire for people battling with one health challenge or the other. What are the physiological effects of low pH on the body organs? Eyes are the first victims of degenerating effects of low pH and its consequences include cataract, glaucoma and other forms of visual impairment. Also, low body pH makes the heart overwork by robbing the blood of proper oxygenation and causing irregular heart beat and systemic degeneration of the heart muscle and blood vessels, which can ultimately lead to heart attack and stroke.

The brain and nerves also malfunction when the body pH is low (acidic pH). Furthermore, acidic pH undermines the vital functions of the pancreas - production of insulin for glucose metabolism and digestive enzymes for synthesis of protein. Yet, the dysfunction of the pancreas triggers diabetes and cancer, with the former setting the stage for the latter. A joint report by the American Cancer

A GUIDE TO A HEALTHIER LIFESTYLE

Society and the American Diabetes Association noted that people with type 2 diabetes have high risk of developing cancers of the liver, pancreas, colon and bladder. Acidic pH causes clogging of the colon with acid wastes resulting in chronic constipation, which makes healing of any health challenge impossible.

Yetunde's TIPS for Healthy alternatives to wheat

* Yam & yam flour

* Unpolished rice

* Sweet potato

* Corn

* Coco yam

* Quaker Oats

P.S Please note that the wheat we eat in this present day is different to that which we ate in the past.

Most wheat grains have genetically modified ingredients in them.

It is time to go back to our roots with naturally grown foods.

YOUR LAUNCH PROGRAMME

If you decide to embark on a "launch" or detox programme, I suggest you choose a week to do this.

You can call it a seven day detoxification time.

During this time, you begin to incorporate Raw Foods into your diet.

Example of the Launch programme will be:

A DAY'S MENU

On waking: drink two large cups of warm water with few drops of lemon or lime or fresh mint tea.

Breakfast: A smoothie made up of freshly made fruits and vegetables. (See Recipe section)

Mid-morning: A freshly made juice

Afternoon: A smoothie or a salad (no- salad cream)

Mid-afternoon: A freshly made fruit and vegetable juice

Dinner: A freshly made Soup.

You will find pointers for recipe ideas in in the Recipe Section.

While on the "launch/detox programme, you can snack on freshly prepared fruits and vegetables like carrots, celery, pears and apples.

Caffeine free teas are the best to take especially during the detox programme and as you continue on the healthy lifestyle journey.

PLEASE NOTE:

Keep a record of what you eat. Either in a notebook or on a calendar on the wall in your kitchen.

You can use fresh lime drops in the place of fresh lemon drops in your water.

After the "launch/detox" week, you can incorporate the "familiar tastes" foods I ate as I embarked on my raw lifestyle journey. See pages 20 - 23.

Also if you do not have all the ingredients readily available, you can improvise.

A GUIDE TO A HEALTHIER LIFESTYLE

A FINAL WORD

You can be the person God wants you to be. You can be the healthy person God wants you to be.

You can be your ideal weight.

It is very important that you do not see this as a diet but as a lifestyle change. This is because if you see at as a diet it is bound to fail. If this journey is perceived as a lifestyle change, it will be easy to keep to.

A lifestyle change means you will be able to run up the stairs, run for the bus, play games/football with a young one without being out of breathe. This will only be do-able if you so decide firstly in your heart that you can do it. That decision however lies with you.

The journey of a thousand miles starts with the first step.

Remember that we do not all have to be a size zero, not everyone has to have a slim waist, the most important thing is that we are healthy enough to live our life to the fullest.

Living your life to the fullest means you are able to help yourself and to help others.

Remember:

- You can do all this through Christ who strengthens YOU!' Phillipians 4:13

- 'Little by little I will drive them out before you, until you are increased and possess the land' Exodus 23:30

YES YOU CAN! GO RAW!

'When there is a will, there is a way'

LOSE WEIGHT, STAY HEALTHY, GAIN LIFE!!!

> 'Most people work hard and spend their health trying to achieve wealth. Then they retire and spend their wealth trying to get back their health.'

It's not a DIET, It's a LIFESTYLE change!

A GUIDE TO A HEALTHIER LIFESTYLE

NEXT STEPS

Dear Reader

Thank you for buying and reading this book. Please look out for more books, as I am still writing and there will be more to follow.

If you have enjoyed this book and have been blessed by reading it, please share and get a copy for your loved ones.

I am available for one to one coaching sessions.

Contact me on www.yetundedaramola.com

www.rawfoods4life.com

Facebook: Yetunde Odebiyi.

Facebook Group: Raw Foods for a Healthier Lifestyle

I also hold seminars. Yetunde welcomes the opportunity to share her experience and offer counselling sessions in your church, in conferences, in retreats, in men's, women's and youth groups.

Your views are very important, so please kindly leave a review online after reading this book.

The Books that changed my way of thinking and helped me on this journey

The Hallelujah Diet by George Malkmus. Once I started reading this book, I could not put it down. I loved the scriptural references and wondered why I had never come across this book. However, due to the fact that it was a book written by an American, most of the ingredients were not readily available in the UK, so I could not try a lot of the recipes. I however, enjoyed the book as it was a complete eye-opener on my Raw Foods and healthy lifestyle journey.

Juice Yourself Slim by Jason Vale. This book became my third bible. It lives in my kitchen and now has a lot of "fresh juice and soup" marks on it. Apart from some of the language in the book, I gained a lot from the book and it helped me on exploring the tastes which I was able to adapt for my own use. The Launch programme was something to "live for". Exactly as it said – Lose 7lbs in 7 days. I "fell in love" with fresh home-made juices, smoothies and soups – even the "bland tasting" ones. Jason surely deserves the title "The juice Master"

Eating Without Heating: Favourite Recipes from Teens Who Love Raw Foods by Sergei Boutenko. Great book with easy to manage many recipes. Most of the ingredients can be found in grocery store. The writers take us through their raw food journey including how they were able to manage Asthma and Diabetes simply by changing their diet. – They are "raw vegetarians" though.

SHORT AND SHARP JUICING TIPS

By Yetunde Odebiyi

This is a self-help book that will be a breeze to get through.

It will be a mini –manual that will complement any kitchen.

I went to visit a friend of mine and her daughter said "Aunty Yetty, I've just made a juice, would you like some? I know you'll like that. "What's in it?" I said. Banana, kiwi, apple, the young lady replied. "I've been juicing everyday".

Aargh, I said, "Sweetheart that is just sugar, where are the vegetables? Her reply: "I did not know I had to add vegetables to my smoothies. No wonder I am not losing any weight".

"We need a shorter and sharper book"…her Mum chipped in.

This book, as the title denotes will go straight to the point of juicing and your taste buds will thank you also.

Coming out soon, for you to enjoy and it will certainly change your life for the better.

Still Not Sure?

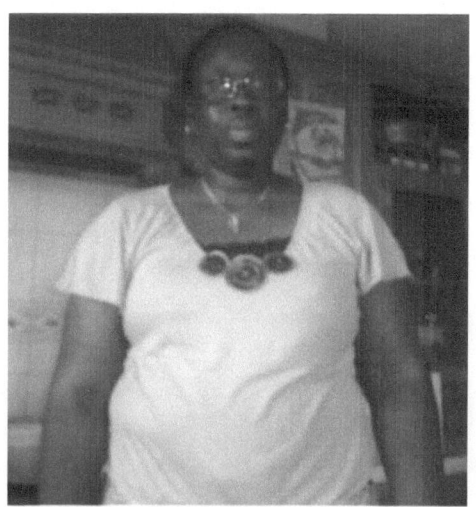

My Heaviest January 2009 (101kgs/15.90 stones/222.63 lbs)

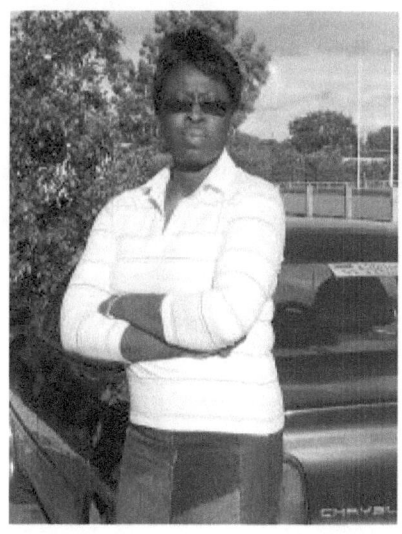

My lightest June 2009 (80kgs/ 12.60 stones/176.37 lbs)

YOUR NOTES

A GUIDE TO A HEALTHIER LIFESTYLE